March, 2007

Janis –

Best wishes in Nursing education!

Linda Caputi

Little Lessons for Nurse Educators

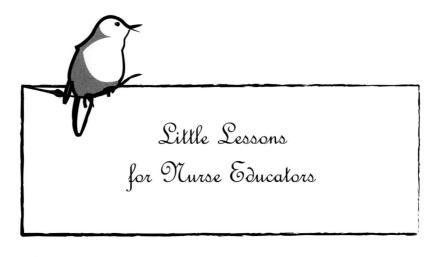

Little Lessons
for Nurse Educators

by Linda Caputi, RN, MSN, EdD, CNE

College of DuPage Press

Little Lessons for Nurse Educators
By Linda Caputi, RN, MSN, EdD, CNE
College of DuPage Press
Glen Ellyn, Illinois
© 2007, College of DuPage Press

Text copyright © 2007 by Linda Caputi, RN, MSN, EdD, CNE

Book cover and design by Janice Walker

Caputi, Linda.
  Little lessons for nurse educators / by Linda Caputi.
      p. ; cm.
  Includes bibliographical references.
  ISBN-13: 978-1-932514-13-1 (alk. paper)
  ISBN-10: 1-932514-13-9 (alk. paper)
  1. Nursing--Study and teaching. I. Title.
  [DNLM: 1. Education, Nursing. 2. Philosophy. WY 18 C255L 2007]
  RT71.C425 2007
  610.73071'1--dc22
                              2006030543

This book is dedicated to all nursing faculty and all nursing students everywhere.
- Linda Caputi, RN, MSN, EdD, CNE

As nurses, we know who we are. The American Nurses Association and other groups have skillfully defined nursing. We are familiar with those definitions and identify with them in our practice as nurses. We have applied those definitions to the real world and know ourselves as nurses within those frameworks.

As nursing faculty, our self-concept may be a bit fuzzier. It has only been recently that the National League for Nursing (2005) has developed the eight core competencies for nurse educators included in *The Scope of Practice for Academic Nurse Educators*. This document provides a formal framework for nursing faculty to understand their roles and responsibilities, but it is only a beginning.

While this framework is important to helping us craft our self-concept as educators, we each must build a personal philosophy of teaching. Teaching is very personal and is as unique to all of us as our personalities.

I discovered this uniqueness in personal teaching philosophy when putting together the first three volumes of *Teaching Nursing: The Art and Science*. I asked each contributor to include with their chapter a brief statement about their philosophy of teaching. There were sixty-one contributors and each philosophy statement was unique. I had expected more likeness in these faculty statements. I shouldn't have been surprised –I know from my own colleagues how different our approaches to teaching can be.

This rich diversity started me on the road to this little book. It is my intent to provide insights, illustrations, inspirations, and reflections to help us define ourselves as teachers and assist in our quest to build a personal philosophy of nursing education. On another level, I hope this book will not only provide some understanding of ourselves as the teachers we are now, but more importantly, *the teachers we might become.*

Understanding ourselves and our philosophy of teaching does more than give us self knowledge. This understanding also:

- Offers a way to understand others, to appreciate the many perspectives on teaching our colleagues have and to minimize conflict and help us work together effectively.
- Gives us a set of values to facilitate adopting new learning strategies and teaching ideas.
- Promotes confidence in our own abilities.
- Provides a source of continuity and stability in times of change or crisis.

I hope this little book will help us all – new and experienced teachers – on the path toward a clearer definition of our own educational philosophy.

- L. C.

This book is formatted simply. It presents a quote then applies that quote's message to lessons for nursing education. Each little lesson is closed with a "Nightingale," a succinct statement or useful hint to epitomize the idea.

I call these succinct statements "Nightingales" as a tribute to Florence Nightingale, the first nurse educator, who when she returned from the Crimean War, in 1856 sought the "…establishment of a school for nurses" (NLN, 2005, p. 3). I use the illustration of the bird, the nightingale, whose sweet song is symbolic of the voice of Florence as she called for the education of nurses. I offer this book to her memory.

I do not pretend to teach her [the nurse] how, I ask
her to teach herself, and for this purpose I venture to
give her some hints.
- Florence Nightingale, Notes on Nursing, 1859

What a humble woman! At the time Florence Nightingale – the first nurse researcher, the first nurse educator – knew more about nursing than any one else, yet she gave herself credit for only giving "some hints," and the nurse will teach "herself." Ms. Nightingale understood the need for education and the need for students to be active in their learning.

Perhaps this is what we do as teachers. Active learning theory explains that students must be actively engaged in learning. Through this active process, they are learning to teach themselves, building on what we have taught. This is an extremely valuable skill to learn. Consider the information we are teaching. That information becomes outdated at a faster rate each year than the year before. Perhaps we are doing as Florence did, we are giving hints when we teach, and the real teaching lies within the student. This sets the stage for life-long learning, a critical aspect of a professional. Nurses continually teach themselves as they remain competent in their specialty areas. Our learning is never finished.

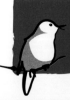

Smart, prophetic, and humble; those are the characteristics of our first nurse educator, our first nursing faculty role model.

Movement toward excellence and innovation is achieved and sustained when there are people who strive to be the very best they can be – and do the very best they can – because they cannot imagine functioning in any other way. We encourage you to think about what excellence in nursing education means to you and your school and then to take the risks associated with persistently moving toward it.

- Pamela M. Ironside and
Theresa M. Valiga (Page 121)

Striving to be your best. This is what most nurse educators do. Most nurse educators continue to work toward perfection; it's in their nature. This search for excellence continues throughout the educator's professional career.

I was conducting a workshop for a group of nursing faculty in California. At break a very dignified and elegant attendee approached me. As she smiled, I thought to myself, "Isn't this nice. This lady looks as though she is nearing retirement age, yet she is attending this faculty development workshop." I was impressed. Little did I know how much more impressed I would be at the completion of our conversation.

"Hello, Dr. Caputi. You offer some wonderful ideas to use in the classroom," she said. I thanked her and asked if she teaches only in the classroom or if she also teaches in the clinical area. She replied, "Oh, I am getting a little older these days and find the clinical is a little difficult for me." I asked her how long it had been since she had taught in the clinical (privately calculating how many more years I may have in that very busy environment!). She replied, "Well, that was about 10 years ago. I was 70 at the time."

I was extremely surprised, to say the least! Not only was this person still teaching at 80 years of age, but, by attending the workshop, she was continuing to strive to be the best she can be. What an inspiration!

Always work hungry – to learn, to teach, to move students – no matter how long you've been teaching!

I have not failed.
I've just found 10,000 ways that don't work.
- Thomas Edison

Ever try something new and it didn't work? Did you feel as if you failed? Knowing what doesn't work can be as important as knowing what does work. What not to do is as important as what to do. Learn from this experience; learn what works and learn what doesn't work. But, keep trying. Don't allow an occasional failure to dampen your spirits! Some strategies may not work with your initial implementation. If you believe it is worth revising and retrying, do so. It may need even further tweaking with a third or even fourth implementation. Keep reworking the instructional strategy until it is the best it can be. However, if it just plain doesn't work, then throw it out!

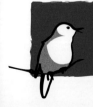

Be ruthless! Keep the best; throw out the rest.

Genius is one percent inspiration and
ninety-nine percent perspiration.
- Thomas Edison

When we see the end product of a great idea, what appears to be effortless genius is actually hard work. Having a great idea is only the beginning. Seeing that idea through to fruition is hard work - and nothing is more off-putting than the four letter word: W-O-R-K!

Be prepared to work when you have a wonderful idea. Others may like your idea, but you are the one who will be expected to stick with the idea to completion. People may even be willing to help you, but you will be the "idea manager," that is, the person who manages the work to ensure the idea comes to life.

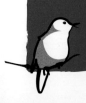 Great idea? Nourish your great idea with hard work.

Student engagement is a key factor in learning. We do not know what is on their minds when they sit down. Our job is to snap them to attention and concentrate it on the topic for the day – to be fully engaged in learning activities.
- Ronald Berk (Page 5)

Students must be engaged in all learning environments. Engage students in the classroom with active learning strategies. Engage students in the nursing laboratory with simulations and contextual return demonstrations of skills. Engage students in the clinical with portfolio development and critical thinking activities. We have little time with students, so have little time to waste.

Engage your students. Passive teaching is no more effective than passive learning.

It is not enough to have a good mind;
the main thing is to use it well.
- Rene Descartes

So what does "to use it well" mean? To "use it well" comes in many forms, such as teaching students to use their minds to manipulate facts and information. It means to identify similarities and differences, differentiate important from unimportant information, and on and on. It means to use knowledge to be knowledgeable; to use critical thinking as the basis for clinical reasoning. It does NOT mean to memorize facts and information.

Using information to be knowledgeable is of major importance in nursing. It is not enough to just know "stuff." The nurse must use information, manipulate it, and apply it to plan patient care – care that not only heals, but care that prevents complications. It is not enough for our graduates to enter the workforce just knowing facts and information. We must teach them to think critically about patient data, what that data mean, and what the nurse does with that information.

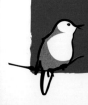

Teach your students to think!

Good teaching is one-fourth preparation
and three-fourths pure theatre.
- Gail Godwin
(Twentieth Century, National Best Seller Author)

Ever wonder why you're so tired after spending a day in the classroom? After all, you're just talking, why should that be so tiring? You're tired because you are on-stage, so to speak. You are expected to perform. Sometimes your performance is scripted, as when you work from prepared notes. Other times your teaching involves improvisation, as when you are leading a discussion or helping students work through a case study.

At all times, you never know what questions your students may ask. There is always the anxiety that a student may ask a question for which you do not have the answer! This anxiety contributes to the fatigue of teaching.

Relax and enjoy your time with students. Know that you will not have all the answers. This is fact. Accept it.

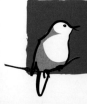

Relax and let your personality and style shine through!

Education is what survives when what
has been learned has been forgotten.
- B. F. Skinner

Much of what students learn will soon be replaced by new information. Think about what you learned in nursing school. How much of that information is still current? In this quote education refers to the process of knowing how to learn, knowing how to solve problems, and knowing where to get needed information. These are intellectual skills we must teach our students so they will be educated and not merely containers of information.

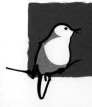

Teach thinking first, then facts.

All men who have turned out worth anything have
had the chief hand in their own education.
- Sir Walter Scott

Although many students may prefer faculty telling them what they need to know, this is not the best way to learn. Students must be active in their learning. Active learning facilitates deeper, more meaningful learning. Students must actively engage in the learning process. Some students enter nursing programs with the skills to actively learn; many do not. It is the teacher's responsibility to design learning strategies so students can experience meaningful learning. Straight lecture cannot be the primary way of teaching. In both the classroom and clinical, the teacher must engage students to be active in their learning. In this way, students learn how to learn. Teaching learning strategies while teaching content empowers the student to succeed.

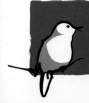

Learning is active.

Keep away from people who try to belittle your ambitions. Small people always do that, but the really great make you feel that you, too, can become great.
- Mark Twain

There will be times in the life of all nurse educators when they attend a conference or workshop, learn something absolutely intriguing, and enthusiastically share that new idea with their colleagues. Some of those colleagues will belittle the idea and discourage its use. The enthusiastic teacher may hear comments such as, "We already tried that." Or, "That will never work."

Maybe the idea has been tried; however, times change, students change, the healthcare environment changes, and education changes! Don't let a naysayer discourage you. Thank them for their feedback and forge ahead. Try that new idea! This old Chinese proverb applies here, "The person who says it cannot be done should not interrupt the person doing it."

It is helpful to associate with positive people in the work place who appreciate good teaching and are dedicated faculty. These are the truly great people in your life, supportive people who will help you become a great teacher.

Surround yourself with "great" people – those who encourage you and find value in your work!

She excelled at school, at a time before segregation was fully abolished, and remembers how a white teacher, who had taught her in the sixth to eighth grades, would ask about her progress when she met her in the town and would give her a dollar for her A grades and 50 cents for her Bs. This left a powerful impression on her, to know that someone had an interest and an investment in her and was helping her to move ahead. The importance of mentoring is something which has stayed with her as a theme.
- Professor Liz Meerabeau, Head of School of Health and Social Care, University of Greenwich about Dr. Beverly Malone

What a profound effect a teacher can have! So what happened to this person, Beverly Malone? What did she become? Noting positions of just the last 10 years of her career, the list includes:

- Dean, Interim Vice Chancellor of Academic Affairs and Professor at North Carolina A&T State University, School of Nursing
- President of the American Nurses Association
- Appointed by President Clinton as a member of the U.S. delegation to the World Health Assembly and served as a member of President Clinton's Advisory Commission on Consumer Protection and Quality in the Health Care Industry
- Deputy Assistant Secretary of Heath in the U S. Department of Health and Human Services
- General Secretary of the Royal College of Nursing of the United Kingdom
- CEO of the National League for Nursing (2007)

Mentor your students; they are the nursing leaders of tomorrow!

Insanity: doing the same thing over and over again
and expecting different results.
- Albert Einstein

Do you sometimes hear comments from faculty such as, "The students this year did not score any higher on the fluid and electrolytes (cardiac, high risk pregnancy, insert your favorite topic) test than last year's students!" Or, "I have been teaching neuro for ten years! Students just don't get it, year after year!"

These are what I call "curriculum choke points." Curriculum choke points are areas of the curriculum that are traditionally difficult for students. Curriculum choke points may be content areas in theory or practice areas in the clinical. Faculty continue to teach the same way and are surprised when the students in the current year "aren't doing any better than last year or the year before!"

Why keep teaching the same topic in the same way and expect different results? Faculty must take ownership of this situation. This is not the students' problem. Faculty much change the way they teach these "choke points" and find a different way, a way that works so students can learn.

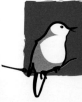

Set solid goals for student performance and improve your
teaching until those goals are reached.

The power to question is the basis of
all human progress.
- Indira Gandhi

Nursing faculty must learn how to question students. Asking questions is an excellent strategy for fostering critical thinking, which is the basis for clinical reasoning and judgment. When students experience faculty asking them questions about their patient care, students learn to ask questions of themselves. When they enter practice as new graduates, they will be able to identify what questions need answering as they approach patient care. The power to question – that is what moves your students from memorization of facts to application and analysis of data for better patient outcomes.

However, the power to question is a learned skill. Teachers must be knowledgeable about the *kinds* of questions to ask and *how* to ask those questions. Questions should progress from easy to difficult. For example, as the teacher interacts with a student in the clinical, the teacher asks a question about basic care the student will provide. If the student can answer that question, then a higher-level question is asked. This questioning continues as the teacher explores the student's ability to engage in more complex thinking.

Asking questions fosters critical thinking – the basis for clinical judgment! Learn how to ask questions.

There are two kinds of people, those who do the work and those who take the credit. Try to be in the first group; there is less competition there.
- Indira Gandhi

There is indeed less competition to be a member of the "work" group, but those who do the work should get the credit. It is difficult to have a culture of collegiality when someone takes the credit for someone else's work. Even more disconcerting is when one faculty works very hard to accomplish a task or goal for the good of the group and no recognition is given to that person. The spirit dies. The spark and zest which fuels creative work soon dies and is replaced with disappointment. This is disastrous for both the individual faculty and the faculty group.

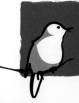

Don't be shy – take credit for what you accomplish and give credit to others for their accomplishments.

It requires the same energy to laugh as it does to cry –
and laughing is a lot more fun.
- Tim Porter-O'Grady (Page 4)

29

Enjoy yourself! Your love for your profession is contagious. Students will experience your enjoyment and your enthusiasm and learn to love nursing as you do. Incorporating appropriate use of humor into your teaching can help in many ways. For example, humor:

1. Transforms abstract concepts into visual events; visual events are remembered longer than the spoken word alone.
2. Enhances memory, retention, and recall.
3. Arouses attention and interest.
4. Enhances self-esteem.
5. Reduces stress.
6. Enhances creative thinking.
7. Enriches the student-teacher relationship.

Humor, when used appropriately, is a sound instructional strategy. Some people contend that they are not in the classroom to entertain, but to teach. As is apparent throughout this book, teaching takes many forms. This particular form of teaching is known as "edutainment."

Lighten up! Use edutainment in your teaching as a planned instructional strategy to help students learn and enhance recall of that learning at a later time.

I dwell in possibility.
- Emily Dickinson

Dwell in possibility! What a wonderful thought! We must believe that what we aspire to do is possible. Our plans to improve our teaching are possible. Perhaps not in their first or second forms, but with revision, ideas can be molded into viable realities. A positive attitude is an absolute necessity for turning possibilities into reality.

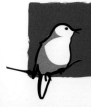

Dwell in possibility.

Curriculum is the interactions and transactions that occur between and among students and teachers with the intent that learning occur. (Page 5) This learning must illuminate, must awaken, must liberate the human mind and harness its potential. And when viewed this way, the key element of the whole is not in the philosophy of the school, not in the curriculum plan or the program of studies, nor in the design of the buildings and grounds and the richness of the equipment, but in the quality of teaching, the imagination of the faculty for designing and selecting learning activities, and in how faculty interact with students.

- Ema Olivia Bevis and Jean Watson (Page 164)

This approach to curriculum is profound in that it puts the onus of responsibility on the individual teacher. It also explains an experience I had as a new teacher. I remember delivering content in the lecture format. The lecture was organized, clearly delivered, and well received by the students. The test was largely composed of application and analysis level questions. When one student turned in her test she remarked, "I'm a second-career student. In my first career I was a teacher. I see that you teach at the knowledge/comprehension level but test at the application/analysis level. That's really not fair to the student. I didn't expect this." She was so right!

What Bevis and Watson propose is exactly what the student was suggesting. Curriculum is all about the interaction between faculty and students. The way one teaches determines the type of nurse the student becomes, and that's the purpose of a curriculum. Does the curriculum produce a nurse who has memorized facts about nursing care and procedures for nursing skills? Or, does the curriculum produce a nurse with a liberated mind to consider alternatives and engage in critical thinking?

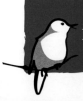
Plan your curriculum for the type of nurse you want to educate.

Give the best educational experience possible. I feel faculty should continuously challenge themselves to provide creative, interesting, and sound education – students soon learn that education doesn't have to be boring; they become self-motivated, enthusiastic, and interested...learning then follows.
- Linda Caputi (Page 2)

As a new teacher many years ago, I recall lecturing to a group of 60 students. Looking at the students during lecture I noticed glazed eyes, yawns, and even a few heads resting on folded arms on the desk. I, myself, was actually a little bit bored and felt like napping, except I was expected to continue "teaching" until the end of the class time. This had to change!

Several years later I attended a conference where Patty Wooten was talking about using humor in education. I was just given permission to laugh in the classroom! I immediately wanted to learn more! I returned home and began researching the topic of appropriate use of humor in the classroom. Soon my classroom teaching included top 10 lists, funny songs, raps for review, and even a dance or two. Class was no longer boring. In fact, there have been several occasions when students attending a morning class returned for the repeated session for the afternoon class. When I asked why they returned, they merely replied that they enjoyed class and wanted a repeat session. What a compliment!

Allen Funt from *Candid Camera* once said, "When people are smiling they are most receptive to almost anything you want to teach them." I believe that quote applies here.

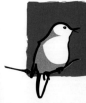

Make learning fun; it doesn't have to be boring!

One moment of patience may ward off great disaster.
One moment of impatience may ruin a whole life.
- Chinese Proverb

As a nurse educator you are very busy. Some of your busiest times may well be when supervising students in the clinical experience when you feel as though demands are coming at you from all directions. Students need you to:

- Administer medications
- Perform dressing changes
- Discharge a patient
- Perform patient teaching
- On and on and on

Students, by their very nature, perform these interventions much slower than the licensed nurses. You must not be impatient. Have compassion for your novice learner. Allow students a reasonable amount of time to provide patient care. If you find you do not have enough time to provide the supervision necessary, as well as time for both teaching and evaluating, then rethink your approach to clinical instruction. Clinical is a classroom and you are in control and responsible for arranging learning experiences for your students.

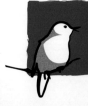

Without compassion and patience, no teaching
should take place.

Right now I'm faced with a task that is not my forte.
But I always tell myself, if someone else can do this,
so can you!
- Dr. Ruena Norman, Interim Director of Nursing,
Florida A&M University, Tallahassee, Florida

I was recently invited to conduct a faculty workshop at Florida A&M University (FAMU) in Tallahassee, Florida. As I waited for a connecting flight in Raleigh, North Carolina, I found myself sitting next to a young lady with a tote bag from a nurse practitioner conference. We started talking and I mentioned I was on my way to conduct a workshop for the FAMU nursing faculty. The young lady exclaimed, "Oh! You'll meet Dr. Norman! She was my professor and such an inspiration to me. I am now an adjunct faculty at FAMU and Dr. Norman continues to inspire me."

After I arrived in Tallahassee and met Dr. Norman, I quickly realized why this young nurse was inspired. Spending only a few minutes with Dr. Norman was all that was needed to detect her positive, can-do attitude, as exemplified in the quote. Her personality exudes her nature as a positivist. I knew immediately that I would have a good workshop with her faculty just from her attitude! What a joy to be in her presence.

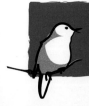

Give your students the gift of a positive attitude!

One's mind, once stretched by a new idea, never
regains its original dimensions.
- Oliver Wendell Holmes

Stretch your students' minds. Challenge them with case studies, simulations, concept mapping, and an array of other learning strategies. Use active learning as much as possible. Make students think about what you are teaching, not merely memorize the information you are providing.

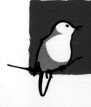

Engage your students in exercises that stretch their minds!

Learning is an activity that cannot be shared, but is rather the responsibility of the learner, it is the teacher's responsibility to seek the best possible negotiation of meanings and an emotional climate that is conducive to learn meaningfully. In my experience, most teachers, especially novice teachers, focus on teaching activities and tend to ignore learning activities.
- Joseph D. Novak (Page 113)

Over the last decade there has been a paradigm shift from a teacher-centered classroom to a learner-centered classroom. Educators such as Dr. Novak have provided effective learning strategies to engage students in meaningful learning. Dr. Novak developed the concept map which is used extensively in nursing education.

Meaningful learning refers to students learning information, then using that information in some meaningful way. In this manner, students become knowledgeable about a discipline rather than simply memorizing the information of that discipline.

Encourage meaningful learning; discourage rote memorization.

Expertise takes time to develop and it is neither cost-effective nor practical to try to "teach" it in formal educational programs.
- Patricia Benner (Page 184)

Dr. Benner helped nurse educators realize that our students will not be experts when they leave us. Upon graduation students have reached the advanced beginner stage. Nursing faculty must accept this and write program outcomes that reflect realistic expectations. We must know about our learners, where they are in their learning, and their characteristics at every stage. We must know where they start and plan a realistic level for them to achieve when they finish the nursing program. These are the outcomes we must identify for our students.

It is time for nursing education programs and the clinical practice settings to collaborate. This collaboration is crucial because the practice setting takes over where education leaves off. Both arenas must have realistic expectations. If there is no collaboration, the new graduate may be expected to perform at an unrealistic level. This will be frustrating for the new nurse and may force the nurse to leave nursing. A strong collaboration between education and practice is the ideal for a smooth and successful transition for the newly-graduated nurse.

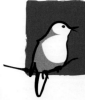

Knowing how a nurse moves from novice to expert empowers you in the classroom.

To repeat what others have said requires learning; to analyze, apply, manipulate, and create requires critical thinking. Nursing students must learn to do the latter.
- Linda Caputi

I recently received a call, similar to calls I receive every year, from a unit manager requesting a reference for one of my students who had applied to work in the Critical Care Unit. She asked me how the student performed while under my watch. I proceeded to tell her what a wonderful student she was…how she could perform all kinds of nursing skills safely and effectively. She responded that she didn't want to know about that; she wanted to know if the student could think.

"Will she be able to solve problems?"

"Will she be prepared to call the physician?"

"Is she a critical thinker?"

I was able to answer a resounding YES!

As nursing faculty, I want a student who can think. I want a student who uses information as a knowledge base for critical thinking that supports clinical judgment. I do not want students to know how to perform tasks, but not know how to think about those tasks. Students of that sort are taskers not thinkers. What kind of student do you want?

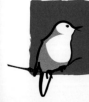

Teach your students to think!

The future ain't what it used to be.
- Yogi Berra, Baseball Great

The future will come, and it is likely to be quite different than the present. How does a nurse educator prepare for the future of nursing? Perhaps it is best to let the future happen and then adjust. However, this may be a costly path to take in terms of time and student preparation. So, how does a nurse educator prepare for the future?

The good news is that you are not alone in planning for the future. There are many organizations working to prepare nursing education for the years ahead. Your responsibility is to keep abreast of the latest ideas from these organizations. Examples of organizations include the National League for Nursing, the American Association of Colleges of Nursing, the National Council of State Boards of Nursing, the National Organization for Associate Degree Nursing, the National Association for Practical Nurse Education and Service, the National Student Nurses' Association, Sigma Theta Tau, and the Joint Commission on Accreditation of Healthcare Organizations. There are many specialty practice organizations as well.

Assign groups of faculty to standing committees with each committee monitoring a specific organization. Each group reports to the full faculty at scheduled meetings and the information is used to update curriculum on an ongoing basis. Become active in these organizations, serve on committees and attend conventions. Use what is learned from these organizations to maintain currency in your nursing program and in your own professional growth.

Use your professional organizations to empower your teaching!

Teaching occurs only when learning takes place.
- Ken Bain (Page 173)

This quote represents a major, but necessary, shift in thinking; almost a paradigm shift! I remember saying, "But I told them that in class! Why didn't they learn?" With this shift in thinking, I will now have to say, "They didn't learn; I must not have taught it."

I may have thought I taught it. I stood in front of the classroom and told the students all about that topic. But telling is not teaching! Telling involves transmitting *information*. Teaching involves transmitting *knowledge* so the student can use that knowledge in a meaningful way.

Teaching is more than just telling. Telling involves no application of learning strategies. Telling is passive, not active, for the student. No matter how interesting the topic may be, there is more to learning than merely listening to a speaker talk about a topic. After all, we only remember 20% of what we hear.

We remember:
- 10% of what we read
- 20% of what we hear
- 30% of what we see
- 50% of what we both see and hear
- 70% of what we discuss
- 80% of what we do/experience
- 90% of what we teach someone else

We must engage students to be actively involved in learning. We must engage students to help them learn. After all, if learning didn't take place, then teaching did not occur.

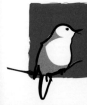

Telling is not teaching.

Go to work smiling.
- Warren Buffet

Go to bed every night looking forward to the excitement of tomorrow. Be excited about spending time with your students, trying a new learning strategy, and even writing a great test! Go to bed with the thought that you can't wait to wake up in the morning because you will be going to school for yet another day with your students. This is exactly how I feel every night. I am blessed. I go to work smiling and plan to do so for a long time to come.

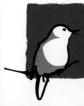

Be excited about tomorrow.

It is not the answer that enlightens, but the question.
- Eugene Ionesco, Romanian Playwright, 1909-1994

Questions come in two forms: questions teachers ask and questions students ask. As teachers, we take pride when we can intelligently and confidently answer a student's question. We take pride in knowing the answers. We sometimes panic if we don't know the answer to a student's question. We feel we must have all the answers.

We must rethink this approach to teaching. We must be comfortable not having all the answers. We must learn when to give an answer and when to ask a question. Students learn from both. And, as the quote tells us, questions enlighten.

Always provide time for students to ask questions. It is often that a teacher does not get a response from students at the end of a class session when the teacher asks, "Are there any questions?" Try rephrasing your question to: "What are your questions?" Or, "What questions do you have that I have left unanswered?" It is important to ask the right question to elicit questions from your students.

We must also ask questions to encourage thinking about the issue at hand. Questions are an excellent way to foster learning. Start a classroom session with questions. Use questions as "advanced organizers," then at the end of the class ask the students if the questions were answered and how they were answered. Continuously ask questions in the clinical. Students can transfer the experience of being asked questions while in school to their professional practice after they graduate. They will use that experience to know what questions to ask of themselves. I have had many students return after graduation and tell me that, after receiving report on their patients, they often ask themselves, "What would Dr. Caputi ask me about these patients? What would be important for me to think about?"

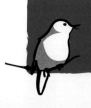

Good questions make good teachers and good learners.

There is no such thing as a bad test question, there are
just some questions that need to be revised.
- Susan Morrison, President of
Health Information Systems, Inc.

Tests are so very important in education. Yet both teachers and students dread their part in the test experience. Think about tests not only as a way to evaluate student learning, but to evaluate your teaching. Use them to identify areas you need to change in your teaching, areas that need more emphasis or a different approach to instruction. Those are the areas that you identify when you are reviewing the results of a test and you say, "My goodness, the students just didn't 'get it'!"

For tests to be useful as indicators of student or teacher performance, they have to be valid and reliable. That is the importance of well-constructed test items. Writing well-constructed test items is the challenge for nursing faculty. Meeting that challenge requires continuous faculty development. The way in which test questions are constructed to evaluate learning is constantly changing. For example, questions are written at higher levels of thinking than in the past, written without bias, and should relate to an area of the NCLEX® test plan. These are only a few of the guidelines that are currently in place, with the promise the future will bring more. Thus, the need exists for continuing education for nurse educators on how to write good test items. Writing good test items doesn't mean throwing out the "bad" ones, it means revising them to comply with the current standards.

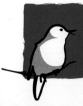

The only thing tougher than answering a good question is writing one.

We teach nursing, we touch the future.
- Gail Baumlein

I once received an email from a student two months after graduation. She had immediately enrolled in a BSN completion program at a state university. Here is what she said:

Hello Linda,

I applied for a full time job in the Emergency Department, which was offered to me, but I am going to turn it down. My professors here want me to get my masters and have been telling me how to prepare for it. I think they really see something in me (not that you didn't!).

I am taking one class this summer and four in the fall. I am really excited and think that I am going to pursue my adult nurse practitioner degree. I have really struggled with this because I don't see myself as smart enough. However, I think I found that thing inside that I have been missing: confidence. Why is it that everyone around me has said how smart I am but yet I struggle to see it? I think it's because I set my goals higher than most so I never see myself as a finished product. The problem is I see my path as just the beginning and fail to recognize exactly how far I have come. My mom says this is classic overachiever-itis. I guess I am starting to see myself as being smart and that does not have to be arrogant. It can just be what it is, and suddenly I feel complete where I am at, even if I have just begun.

I have not felt such peace in a long time. I think it means I am ready, at least that is how I am going to take it. My lightning flash in the sky from God that I have been waiting for has arrived and it feels good.

Thanks for being a sounding board for me. It is good to have such a friend and mentor as you. — Geri Bartnik

This student's story demonstrates how we touch lives, not only when students are in our charge, but potentially for the rest of their lives.

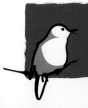

If we could realize how profoundly we affect students' lives, we'd be humbled.

"I want to say is thank you and when I graduate I want to be the kind of nurse you are."
- College of DuPage Nursing Student, 1983, during her final clinical evaluation

The teacher takes the student into the teacher's world of expertise, wisdom, and knowledge. The student learns, grows, and matures, then is released into the world of nursing. When entering this world, the graduate nurse takes some of the teacher along. What will your students take with them? What are you contributing? Just as parents often hear their own words when their adult child speaks, students will repeat what the teacher has spoken. What will your students be saying?

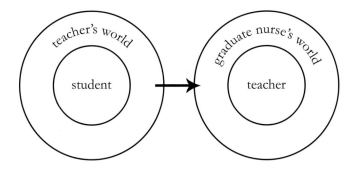

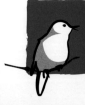

Be proud when you hear your graduates speak.

Teaching in nursing involves the assessment of student learning needs, development of experiences to meet those needs, and evaluation of student achievement. Teaching requires involvement of the learner and a supportive environment in which learning can take place. Teaching strategies in nursing foster development of not only knowledge and skills for practice, but also problem-solving and critical-thinking abilities.
- Marilyn Oermann (Page 126)

In this quote, Dr. Oermann has presented a very succinct description of the instructional design process. It is imperative for nursing faculty to have an understanding of what instructional design is all about and to apply instructional design to their teaching. All faculty are designers of instruction.

A key phrase in Dr. Oermann's quote is "a supportive environment." Instruction is designed to be delivered in a supportive environment. Students need support from faculty. We must provide a caring, supportive environment for students to grow and mature. In turn, students will provide a caring, supportive environment for their patients. This demonstrates how teachers not only touch the lives of their students, but also the lives of all the patients entrusted in the care of their graduates.

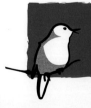

The lives you touch increases exponentially with each and every student you teach.

The teacher who artfully engages students in an atmosphere rich in trust, rapport, and resources is well on the way to developing a climate just right in which to learn. Students need to feel safe to explore and question, in order to gain meaning from their experiences. Students also need focus and perspective. In a collaborative atmosphere, both teacher and student are learners.
- Lynn Engelmann (Page 20)

Your students bring with them rich life and professional experiences. Honor those experiences and the student. As a teacher, you learn from your students.

After teaching for a period of time, you will discover the way you teach students today may not work tomorrow. Why? Because students change, health care changes, and nursing education changes. Learn from your students what works and what doesn't work in the way you are teaching them. Learn to adapt. Learn from your students who *you* are as a teacher.

Do your students respect you? Fear you? Take you seriously? Don't take you seriously? Are they doing well? Doing poorly?

Learn from the looks on their faces in class. Are you boring? Interesting? Confusing? Clear?

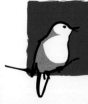

The best teachers learn most from their students.

The more important your cheese is to you the more
you want to hold on to it.
- Spencer Johnson (Page 36)

In the amazing little book *Who Moved My Cheese?*, cheese is a metaphor for what we want in life. For our purposes, cheese is a metaphor for what we want in our faculty position. When we get what we want, we love it and become very comfortable with what we have and how we teach. Then, just when we are totally secure in what we are doing and how we are doing it, someone unexpectedly moves the cheese! How stressful! What do you do? You either move with the cheese or you resist. Moving with the cheese requires energy: energy to learn new things, energy to learn new ways of doing things, energy to replace old teaching strategies with new approaches. To resist also requires energy: energy to maintain the status quo in a changing environment, and energy to defend one's reasons for not changing.

I have found that the energy required to change produces growth, excitement, and renewal. Energy spent resisting change produces wear, tear, and fatigue.

Change happens. Students change, nursing changes, and education changes. Of these three, education is the slowest to change. Occasionally this is good; most times it is not.

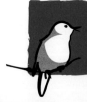

When your cheese moves, move with it.

What has become increasingly apparent to me over the years … is the exceedingly important role that teachers' ego needs play in how they organize the context for learning and how they operate in it. Those teachers who do not have a strong ego perception of "I'm okay" often in subtle or explicit way attack the ego of their students.
- Joseph D. Novak (Page 134)

This quote by Dr. Novak reminded me of a situation I once had with a student. Several years ago I was supervising a student in the clinical giving a subcutaneous injection of insulin. The student aspirated before injecting. When we left the room, I said to the student, "You don't have to aspirate with insulin." The student replied, "That's wrong! We were told in lab to aspirate when giving insulin." I took a deep breath then replied, "I am happy to see that you feel comfortable enough with me to challenge what I say. Here's what I want you to do. I'd like you to read about giving insulin in an adult medical/surgical textbook, in a pediatric textbook, and on various credible websites. Then discuss the administration of insulin with some of the staff nurses and, finally, talk with the diabetes educator. After collecting all that information, let's analyze it to determine best practice for this procedure. Thank you for questioning this practice. We will both learn."

Another approach to this student's challenge may have been to inform her that she is the student and I am the teacher. She is wrong and I am right. However, that approach would only meet my ego needs and would have interfered with a healthy teacher-student relationship.

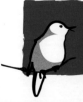

Never let your ego needs interfere with a healthy teacher-student relationship.

For the most part clinical education has remained
essentially unchanged for the past 40 years.
- Christine Tanner (Page 99)

Dr. Tanner explains why the old clinical model must change. To summarize, she notes problems with using the old model:

- Limited number of clinical sites
- Increased patient acuity
- Inefficient use of students' time
- Need for experiences with a variety of patients

She challenges nurse educators to consider new models for clinical instruction. It is imperative that nursing educators in all areas continue this dialogue about clinical teaching and contribute to developing a new model of clinical education. In doing so, faculty must be aware of developments on this topic from organizations such as the National League for Nursing, the American Association of Colleges of Nursing, the American Organization of Nurse Executives, the National Council of State Boards of Nursing, and even the Joint Commission on the Accreditation of Healthcare Organizations. Some of these organizations have crafted position papers on the topic of clinical education, others are researching the topic, and others are providing information about the competencies required of our graduates. We must move ahead.

Be ready to abandon the old modes of clinical education and adopt the new. Or, at the very least, modify.

A teacher decided that a visual demonstration would add emphasis to the topic of the class. The teacher placed four worms into four separate jars.

The first worm was put into a container of alcohol.

The second worm was put into a container of cigarette smoke.

The third worm was put into a container of chocolate syrup.

The fourth worm was put into a container of good, clean soil.

At the conclusion of the lesson, the teacher reported the following results:

The first worm in alcohol - Dead.

The second worm in cigarette smoke - Dead.

The third worm in chocolate syrup - Dead.

The fourth worm in good, clean soil - Alive.

The teacher asked the class, "What can you learn from this demonstration?"

One student quickly raised his hand and said, "As long as you drink, smoke, and eat chocolate, you won't have worms!"

- Anonymous

What an intriguing perspective! The ending was a complete surprise to me and not what I was expecting. This is often what happens when students ask questions – they come as a complete surprise and not what I was expecting! Many times students have intriguing perspectives on a subject that may be quite different than what you are communicating. This is most obvious when discussing test questions! Applaud their creativity and learn from them. They can open your eyes to new ways of thinking.

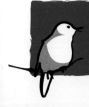

Be prepared for the unexpected!

Gentlemen, this is a football.
- Vince Lombardi, winning coach of the Green Bay
Packers football team

At the beginning of every football season, Vince Lombardi would hold up a football and say to his players, "Gentlemen, this is a football." Seems like an unnecessary statement. These are professional football players who certainly know what a football looks like! Why would he make such a statement? This Super Bowl winning coach did not want his players to ever forget the fundamentals of football.

As faculty, it is easy to get caught up with all that comes our way throughout the school year. These include: efforts to increase NCLEX pass rates, addressing changing accreditation requirements, integrating complex technology into classroom instruction, designing web-based courses, dealing with textbooks that are no longer just textbooks but textbooks with "connections" – connections to web-enhanced and CD-rich resources, not letting budget cuts affect quality education, serving on committees and more committees, and many other responsibilities. Often these distracters can sidetrack faculty from the fundamentals of teaching to the point where we may forget the central component – the student. When feeling overwhelmed and overburdened by all there is to remember, relate, recall, redesign, rewrite, and resubmit, return to the fundamentals of teaching by rephrasing Vince Lombardi's mantra.

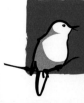

Faculty, this is a student.

You have brains in your head.
You have feet in your shoes.
You can steer yourself
Any direction you choose.
And when things start to happen,
Don't worry. Don't stew.
Just go right along.
You'll start happening, too.
- Dr. Seuss

Choose to follow in the direction of those who love teaching. These teachers are your mentors. They will spark your spirit and give you energy. If you have been teaching for a number of years, be open to new paths. Teaching nursing is an ever-changing specialty. Teachers should not be so entrenched in an idea or a technique that they are unwilling to choose another direction.

When "things" start to happen, you must make a choice. Are "things" happening in the direction you want to take, or are "things" happening in a direction that concerns you? If the case is the former, move in that direction; if the case is the latter, work to move "things" in a better direction.

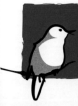

Move in the direction that sparks your spirit for nursing education.

The brain is a beautiful thing. It wakes up with you in
the morning and goes to sleep as soon as you
go to work.
- Robert Frost

This is a very interesting quote! Why would a person's brain go to sleep when that person goes to work? Perhaps the work place forces the person to think in a linear, regimented way. Perhaps creativity isn't rewarded. Perhaps the person is afraid to think "outside of the box." Encourage yourself and those around you to continue to think after arriving at work. Keep your brain working in a creative search for innovative ways to teach your students.

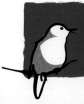

Ruts are everywhere. Nurture your creativity at work; don't allow your work environment to put your brain to sleep!

We all went off to kindergarten with a magical box of
color crayons and graduated from high school with
a disposable ball point pen.
- Maria Girsch and Charlie Girsch (Page 15)

Don't let this trend in education continue in nursing school! Our students must learn to be creative, critical thinkers so they develop their clinical reasoning for better patient outcomes. We cannot continue to stifle their creative spirit by forcing them to memorize information and think in a linear manner. It is our responsibility to teach process so students can apply that process to patient care.

Some studies suggest students are better critical thinkers when they enter nursing school than when they leave nursing school. As nursing faculty, we must stop using teaching strategies that encourage the rote memorization of facts and information and prevent our students from opening their minds to the critical thinking process. We must teach students to be thinkers. We must infuse the curriculum with creative approaches to teaching, such as using concept maps to plan patient care rather than the exclusive use of columnar care plans that results in students copying from textbooks without making critical connections. We must think outside of the box.

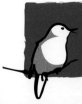

Teach by example; be a role model for creativity and critical thinking.

No, it's not your job.
- Geri Bartnik, College of DuPage graduate,
Class of 2005

In the Fall of 2004, I was teaching a medical-surgical nursing course with a clinical component that met two days a week. About a month into the course, I realized the students were doing quite well. To help them achieve at an even higher level, I decided to focus their learning. My approach was to return home Monday evening, review the evening's activities, and plan an individual approach for each student for their clinical experience on Tuesday. I was excited about the plan.

I instructed the students to meet me in the lobby of the hospital 15 minutes before the start of the clinical time on Tuesday. I took each student aside, provided feedback, and then shared their focus for the day. After talking with the last student, I realized they may have misunderstood my intentions. I explained to them I had reviewed their clinical performance on Monday evening and wanted to provide them with focus and direction so their time spent on Tuesday would be growth-producing for each of them in a very individualized way. They still looked a little puzzled. I thought I would lighten the moment with the comment, "OK, it's my job!" One student surprised me with her response, "No, it's not your job." She paused and said, "It's your passion. We can all see that. You love teaching nursing and helping us become the best nurses we can be. We appreciate that. It's your passion."

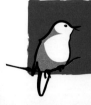

Be passionate about who you teach and what you teach.

Love creates a healing relationship and environment
and laughter cements the two of them together.
- Bernie Siegel, Author of *Love, Medicine & Miracles*

Students of nursing are a very diverse group. They arrive in the classroom with a myriad of prior experiences with education. Many of those experiences may not have been positive. The old adage, "I paid my dues and they must pay theirs" has no place in the current culture of nursing education. This is a dangerous attitude because it clouds thinking and renders the person judgmental.

By providing an educational environment that is caring, faculty create a healing relationship for those students who have been subjected to negativism in previous educational experiences. This is important because students may soon forget what we say, but they will never forget the way we made them feel. Make your students feel good about themselves and their educational experience.

This caring approach to teaching parallels the caring nurses provide for patients. A caring approach to teaching should be mandatory for every nursing curriculum. Once a caring curriculum is established, both teacher and students enjoy their time together as both grow and learn from each other.

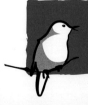

Care about your students and embrace a caring curriculum.

Setting a goal is not the main thing. It is deciding
how you will go about achieving it and
staying with that plan.
- Tom Landry, former head coach of the Dallas
Cowboys football team

Perpetually set goals. Once a goal is achieved, set another. Sometimes these goals are:

- Focused on students, such as goals relating to retention or NCLEX pass rates.
- Related to curriculum, such as goals to integrate more critical thinking into the curriculum or to rewrite the philosophy that guides the curriculum.
- Directed toward professional growth, such as achieving certification as a Certified Nurse Educator or earning a higher degree.

Goals are great; however, goals may remain unrealized if there is no plan for achieving them. People can quickly write goals, but developing a plan and then seeing the plan to fruition is where the difficulty lies. This may be because the goal is set too high and is impossible to achieve. Develop smaller goals that are achievable and eventually lead to accomplishment of a larger goal.

Greatness is but many small steps. Small steps can become great strides on your way to achieving goals.

There are risks and costs to a program of action. But they are far less than the long-range risks and costs of comfortable inaction.
- John F. Kennedy

I recently attended a conference where Dr. Elaine Tagliareni opened with a very interesting keynote. Dr. Tagliareni compared the components of a 1980 curriculum with a 2006 curriculum. As I listened to her compare and contrast, I quickly realized that some of the characteristics of the 1980 curriculum were all too familiar.

The nursing curriculum is a dynamic entity. It must change as nursing students, health care, and educational theory change. This does not need to be a daunting task. As each faculty teaches a course, be alert to what is happening. As faculty attend conferences, information learned should be immediately considered for application to the curriculum. Curriculum revision as an ongoing process is much less painful and more productive than a dreaded task at the end of the school year. An end-of-the-year meeting should be one that integrates the collection of ideas from throughout the year. In the words of Franklin D. Roosevelt, "There are many ways of going forward, but only one way of standing still." The curriculum must move forward.

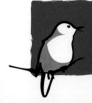

Embrace curriculum change and move forward!

The ultimate measure of a man is not where he stands in moments of comfort, but where he stands at times of challenge and controversy.
- Dr. Martin Luther King, Jr.

These words are applicable when selecting an institutional milieu in which to work. As nursing faculty work through each day, there will be challenges that can stress even the most seasoned (marinated) faculty. Nursing faculty must be assured that as we apply all nursing program policies, adhere to institutional guidelines, and ensure students' rights under applicable laws (such as the Family Educational Rights and Privacy Act [FERPA]), the people who administer the nursing program will support our efforts. There has been an occasional tale from the halls of academia recounting times when faculty have not been supported when difficult decisions are made. Faculty decisions have been reversed for fear of a law suit. Although the faculty's decision may have been the right decision, it was not supported. It may be very uncomfortable to deal with some student situations, but these situations must be handled. If all the right decisions are made, due process provided, and interventions well documented, what must be done must be supported. The nursing profession and patient care are far too important to risk endangerment.

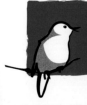

Do the right thing and expect to be supported.

Education has for its object the formation
of character.
- Herbert Spencer English Philosopher (1820 - 1903)

This is so true of nursing! Many students enter the halls of academia with the only image of the nurse being that of the nurse in the current medical television program. This is the basis for their understanding about what a nurse does, how a nurse acts, and what a nurse says. Others arrive with years of experience in other positions in health care, but not from the perspective of a nurse. It is the faculty's responsibility to socialize nursing students into the role of a nurse, building a nursing character.

It is a primary function of the nurse educator to not only serve as teacher, but also serve as role model. Nursing faculty role model the actions of the nurse, the attitude of the nurse, and the professionalism of a nurse. Students take on the character of a nurse primarily from what they learn from their faculty.

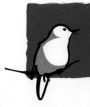

Be true to your profession and proud of the character you build in your students.

In order to further advance nursing education, new models of research-based nursing education must emerge. The precedent of relying on tradition and past practices must be replaced with proposed changes emanating from evidence that substantiates the science of nursing education and provides the foundation for best educational practices.
- National League for Nursing's *The Scope of Practice for Academic Nurse Educators*

The science of nursing education, how exciting! As nursing faculty, we are all given the charge to contribute to the science of nursing education.

Nursing faculty around the country are trying new, exciting, and innovative learning strategies. The problem is, we don't know about them! We must share what we're doing so others can learn about these wonderful strategies. We must research these strategies to determine when to use them, when not to use them, and what modifications can be made for specific populations of students or specific practices areas. We must replace the old "I've always done it that way" methods with research-based best practices. All faculty are called to share their work, to research nursing education, and to share with the broader community of nursing faculty.

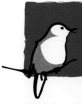
Contribute to the science of nursing education.

We, as teachers, are always becoming and our futures exist as possibilities. Viewed this way, the door is always open to becoming anew.
- Nancy Diekelmann (Page 488)

The time has arrived for all nursing faculty to take stock in what they are doing. Open an honest eye to your teaching practices. Look for those new possibilities Dr. Diekelmann speaks about.

Nursing faculty are the same as all professionals, in that the profession to which we belong is changing. We must accept that we are always becoming and there are so many possibilities that lie ahead.

Dr. Diekelmann is a role model for all nurse educators. She is a trailblazer who has worked many years researching and developing the first pedagogy that is specifically for nursing education. What an achievement! Dr. Diekelmann challenges all nurse educators to build their practice on research and contribute to the science of nursing education. There are so many possibilities yet to be discovered.

No matter your age or years in nursing education, you have only just begun.

And remember, no matter where you go,
there you are.
- Confucius

In other words, no matter where you go in nursing education, there you are. You choose your destination. Will your destination be the status quo or will it be a rewarding profession with exciting adventures in the four scholarships that represent the scholarly work of faculty in schools of nursing? These four scholarships are (Kirkpatrick & Valley, 2004):

- Discovery (Acquisition of new knowledge)
- Integration (Ideas from nursing and other disciplines)
- Application (Clinical practice)
- Teaching (Sharing knowledge)

As you address each of these scholarships in your professional position, enjoy your work. These scholarships represent the milestones on your professional journey, the work in which you engage each day, the "there you are" place on a daily basis. These tasks illuminate your journey and shine your accomplishments. They represent who you are as a professional educator. In other words, they brighten your way as you become who you are as a nurse educator. In the words of Benjamin Franklin, "Hide not your talents. They for use were made. What's a sundial in the shade?"

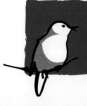

No matter where you go, or at what point you are along the way, "there you are." Enjoy where you are.

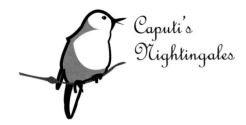

Caputi's Nightingales

1. Smart, prophetic, and humble; those are the characteristics of our first nurse educator, our first nursing faculty role model.

2. Always work hungry – to learn, to teach, to move students – no matter how long you've been teaching!

3. Be ruthless! Keep the best; throw out the rest.

4. Great idea? Nourish your great idea with hard work.

5. Engage your students. Passive teaching is no more effective than passive learning.

6. Teach your students to think!

7. Relax and let your personality and style shine through!

8. Teach thinking first, then facts.

9. Learning is active.

10. Surround yourself with "great" people – those who encourage you and find value in your work!

11. Mentor your students; they are the nursing leaders of tomorrow!

12. Set solid goals for student performance and improve your teaching until those goals are reached.

13. Asking questions fosters critical thinking – the basis for clinical judgment! Learn how to ask questions.

14. Don't be shy – take credit for what you accomplish and give credit to others for their accomplishments.

15. Lighten up! Use edutainment in your teaching as a planned instructional strategy to help students learn and enhance recall of that learning at a later time.

16. Dwell in possibility.

17. Plan your curriculum for the type of nurse you want to educate.

18. Make learning fun; it doesn't have to be boring!

19. Without compassion and patience, no teaching should take place.

20. Give your students the gift of a positive attitude!

21. Engage your students in exercises that stretch their minds!

22. Encourage meaningful learning; discourage rote memorization.

23. Knowing how a nurse moves from novice to expert empowers you in the classroom.

24. Teach your students to think!

25. Use your professional organizations to empower your teaching!

26. Telling is not teaching.

27. Be excited about tomorrow.

28. Good questions make good teachers and good learners.

29. The only thing tougher than answering a good question is writing one.

30. If we could realize how profoundly we affect students' lives, we'd be humbled.

31. Be proud when you hear your graduates speak.

32. The lives you touch increases exponentially with each and every student you teach.

33. The best teachers learn most from their students.

34. When your cheese moves, move with it.

35. Never let your ego needs interfere with a healthy teacher-student relationship.

36. Be ready to abandon the old modes of clinical education and adopt the new. Or, at the very least, modify.

37. Be prepared for the unexpected!

38. Faculty, this is a student.

39. Move in the direction that sparks your spirit for nursing education.

40. Ruts are everywhere. Nurture your creativity at work; don't allow your work environment to put your brain to sleep!

41. Teach by example; be a role model for creativity and critical thinking.

42 Be passionate about who you teach and what you teach.

43. Care about your students and embrace a caring curriculum.

44. Greatness is but many small steps. Small steps can become great strides on your way to achieving goals.

45. Embrace curriculum change and move forward!

46. Do the right thing and expect to be supported.

47. Be true to your profession and proud of the character you build in your students.

48. Contribute to the science of nursing education.

49. No matter your age or years in nursing education, you have only just begun.

50. No matter where you go, or at what point you are along the way, "there you are." Enjoy where you are.

Epilogue

Fifty quotations. Does that cover all the lessons for nurse educators? I would think not. Consider the volumes that have been written about nursing education. The teaching-learning process in nursing education is too complex to be reduced to a list of 50 "Caputi Nightingales." There are many more that can be added and many new ones that will be developed in the future based on changes that will occur in all aspects of nursing education. My hope is that this book has offered enough thought-provoking ideas in its 50 lessons to lead you to an understanding of yourself and your philosophy of teaching.

So, rather than this the end of the book, it is just the beginning.

References

Anderson, L., & Krathwohl, D. (2001). *A taxonomy for learning teaching and assessing: A revision of Bloom's taxonomy of educational objectives.* New York: Longman.

Bain, K. (2004). *What the best college teachers do.* Cambridge, MA: Harvard University Press.

Benner, P. (2001). *From novice to expert: Excellence and power in clinical nursing practice.* (Commemorative ed.). Upper Saddle River, NJ: Prentice Hall.

Bevis, E. O., & Watson, J. (2000). *Toward a caring curriculum: A new pedagogy for nursing.* Boston: Jones and Bartlett.

Berk, R. A. (2002). *Humor as an instructional defibrillator: Evidence-based techniques in teaching and assessment.* Sterling, VA: Stylus.

Caputi, L. (2004). An overview of the educational process. In L. Caputi & L. Engelmann, (Ed.), *Teaching nursing: The art and science. Vols. 1 & 2.* Glen Ellyn, IL: College of DuPage Press.

Caputi, L., & Engelmann, L. (2007, in press) *Teaching nursing: The art and science: Vol. 4.* Glen Ellyn, IL: College of DuPage Press.

Diekelmann, N. (2005). Teacher talk: New pedagogies for nursing. *Journal of Nursing Education, 44*(11), 485-488.

Engelmann, L. (2004). So you're a teacher: Now what do you do? In L. Caputi & L. Engelmann, (Ed.), *Teaching nursing: The art and science. Vols. 1 & 2.* Glen Ellyn, IL: College of DuPage Press.

Girsch, M., & Girsch, C. (1999). *Fanning the creative spirit.* Chicago: CreativityCentral.com.

Ironside, P. M. & Valiga, T. M. (2006). Creating a vision for the future of nursing education: Moving toward excellence through innovation. *Nursing Education Perspectives, 27* (3), 120-121.

Johnson, S. (1998). *Who Moved My Cheese?* New York: Putnam's Sons.

Kirkpatrick, J., & Valley, J. (2004). Finding success in the faculty role. In L. Caputi & L. Engelmann, (Ed.), *Teaching nursing: The art and science. Vols. 1 & 2.* Glen Ellyn, IL: College of DuPage Press.

Meerabeau, L. (2005). http://www.gre.ac.uk/schools/health/eulogy.htm

Morris, S. (2004).Test construction and analysis: Can I do it? In L. Caputi & L. Engelmann, (Eds.), *Teaching nursing: The art and science. Vols. 1 & 2.* Glen Ellyn, IL: College of DuPage Press.

National League for Nursing. (2005). *The Scope of Practice for Academic Nurse Educators.* New York: Author.

Novak, D. J. (1998). *Learning, creating, and using knowledge: Concept maps as facilitative tools in schools and corporations.* Mahwah, NJ: Lawrence Erlbaum.

Oermann, M. (2005). Writing for publication in nursing: What every nurse educator needs to know. In L. Caputi (Ed.), *Teaching nursing: The art and science. Vol.3.* Glen Ellyn, IL: College of DuPage Press.

Palmer, P. (1998). *The courage to teach: Exploring the inner landscape of a teacher's life.* San Francisco: Jossey-Bass.

Porter-O'Grady, P. (1999). Laughter lightens our load. *Nursing Management, 30*(9), 4.

Tanner, C. (2006). The next transformation: Clinical education. *Journal of Nursing Education,45*(4), 99-100.